New Diverticulitis Cookbook for Beginners

New Diverticulitis Cookbook for Beginners

75 Easy High-Fiber and Low-Residue Recipes for Managing Your Health

Avery Bennett

Hopliv Publisher

CONTENTS

1. Introduction 1
2. Understanding Diverticulitis 4
3. High-Fiber Recipes for Non-Flare-Up Periods 7
4. Low-Residue Recipes for Flare-Up Periods 33
5. Weekly Meal Plans 50
6. Lifestyle Tips for Managing Diverticulitis 56
7. Conclusion 58

Copyright © 2024 by Avery Bennett

All rights reserved. No part of this book may be reproduced in any manner whatsoever without written permission except in the case of brief quotations embodied in critical articles and reviews.

First Printing, 2024

1

Introduction

Welcome to the "New Diverticulitis Cookbook for Beginners"! If you're reading this, you or someone you care about is likely dealing with Diverticulitis, a condition that can be both painful and challenging to manage. But don't worry—you've come to the right place. This cookbook is designed to help you navigate your dietary needs with ease, offering delicious and nutritious recipes tailored for every stage of your journey with Diverticulitis.

What is Diverticulitis?

Diverticulitis occurs when small, bulging pouches (diverticula) in the digestive tract become inflamed or infected. These pouches are common, especially after age 40, and don't usually cause problems. However, when they do become inflamed, they can cause severe abdominal pain, fever, nausea, and a significant change in your bowel habits.

Why Diet Matters

Managing Diverticulitis is closely linked to your diet. During non-flare-up periods, a high-fiber diet can help keep your digestive system running smoothly and prevent future flare-ups. However, during a flare-up, a low-residue (low-fiber) diet is essential to minimize irritation and allow your digestive system to heal.

About This Cookbook

This cookbook is divided into two main sections: High-Fiber Recipes for Non-Flare-Up Periods and Low-Residue Recipes for Flare-Up Periods. We've included 75 carefully crafted recipes that are not only good for your gut but also delicious and easy to prepare. Whether you're looking for a hearty breakfast, a light lunch, a satisfying dinner, or a tasty snack, you'll find plenty of options here to suit your needs.

Personal Journey

As someone who has battled Diverticulitis myself, I understand the challenges that come with this condition. I've spent countless hours in the kitchen experimenting with different recipes, searching for meals that are both comforting and kind to my digestive system. Through trial and error, I've discovered a variety of dishes that have helped me feel better and enjoy food again. My hope is that this cookbook will do the same for you.

Getting Started

Before diving into the recipes, I recommend taking a moment to read through the Understanding Diverticulitis chapter. It will provide you with a solid foundation of knowledge about the condition and how diet plays a crucial role in managing it. From there, you can explore the high-fiber and low-residue recipes, as well as weekly meal plans designed to make your life easier.

Remember, managing Diverticulitis is a journey, and you don't have to do it alone. With the right information and the right recipes, you can take control of your health and enjoy delicious meals that nourish your body and soul. So grab your apron, and let's get cooking!

2

Understanding Diverticulitis

What is Diverticulitis?

Diverticulitis is a digestive condition that occurs when small, bulging pouches—known as diverticula—form in the lining of your digestive system and become inflamed or infected. These pouches are most commonly found in the lower part of the large intestine (colon). While diverticula are quite common, especially after the age of 40, they don't usually cause problems. However, when one or more of these pouches become inflamed, the condition is called diverticulitis.

Symptoms of Diverticulitis

The symptoms of diverticulitis can vary from mild to severe. Common symptoms include:

- **Abdominal Pain**: Typically on the lower left side, though it can occur on the right side as well.
- **Fever**: Often accompanies an infection.
- **Nausea and Vomiting**: Due to the body's reaction to the inflammation.
- **Changes in Bowel Habits**: Such as constipation or diarrhea.
- **Bloating**: Feeling of fullness or swelling in the abdomen.

Causes and Risk Factors

The exact cause of diverticulitis is not well understood, but several factors may contribute to the development of the condition:

- **Diet Low in Fiber**: A low-fiber diet can lead to constipation, increasing pressure on the colon walls, which may result in the formation of diverticula.
- **Age**: The risk of diverticulitis increases with age.
- **Obesity**: Being overweight can increase the risk of developing diverticulitis.
- **Smoking**: Smokers are at higher risk.
- **Lack of Exercise**: Regular physical activity can help reduce the risk.
- **Certain Medications**: Including steroids, opioids, and NSAIDs.

The Role of Diet in Managing Diverticulitis

Diet plays a crucial role in both preventing and managing diverticulitis. Here's how:

- **High-Fiber Diet**: During non-flare-up periods, a high-fiber diet helps keep the digestive system functioning smoothly, reducing the risk of constipation and pressure on the colon walls. Foods rich in fiber include fruits, vegetables, whole grains, and legumes.
- **Low-Residue Diet**: During flare-up periods, a low-residue diet is recommended. This diet reduces the amount of undigested food passing through the intestines, minimizing irritation and allowing the digestive system to heal. Low-residue foods include white bread, white rice, and well-cooked vegetables without skins or seeds.

How This Cookbook Can Help

This cookbook provides a collection of recipes specifically designed to help you manage your diet during both flare-up and non-flare-up periods. You'll find:

- **High-Fiber Recipes**: To keep your digestive system healthy and reduce the risk of flare-ups.
- **Low-Residue Recipes**: To soothe your digestive system during flare-ups and promote healing.
- **Weekly Meal Plans**: To simplify your meal planning and ensure you're getting the right nutrients at the right times.

By following the recipes and meal plans in this cookbook, you can take an active role in managing your Diverticulitis, improving your overall health, and enjoying delicious, satisfying meals.

3

High-Fiber Recipes for Non-Flare-Up Periods

High-fiber diets are essential in keeping your digestive system running smoothly and preventing future flare-ups. Here are 40 delicious and nutritious high-fiber recipes to enjoy during non-flare-up periods.

Breakfast Recipes

1. **High-Fiber Oatmeal with Fruits and Nuts**

    - **Ingredients:**
        - 1 cup rolled oats
        - 2 cups water or milk
        - 1 banana, sliced
        - 1/2 cup mixed berries
        - 1/4 cup chopped nuts (almonds, walnuts)
        - 1 tablespoon chia seeds
        - Honey or maple syrup to taste
    - **Instructions:**
        1. Bring the water or milk to a boil in a pot.
        2. Add the rolled oats and reduce the heat to a simmer. Cook for about 5 minutes, stirring occasionally.

3. Top with banana slices, mixed berries, chopped nuts, and chia seeds.
4. Drizzle with honey or maple syrup if desired. Serve warm.

2. **Green Smoothie Bowl**

    - Ingredients:
        - 1 banana
        - 1/2 cup spinach
        - 1/2 cup kale
        - 1/2 avocado
        - 1 cup almond milk
        - 1 tablespoon chia seeds
        - 1/4 cup granola
        - 1/4 cup sliced strawberries
    - Instructions:
        1. Blend the banana, spinach, kale, avocado, almond milk, and chia seeds until smooth.
        2. Pour into a bowl and top with granola and sliced strawberries.

3. **Chia Seed Pudding with Berries**

    - Ingredients:
        - 1/4 cup chia seeds
        - 1 cup almond milk
        - 1 tablespoon honey
        - 1/2 cup mixed berries
    - Instructions:
        1. Mix the chia seeds, almond milk, and honey in a bowl.
        2. Refrigerate for at least 4 hours or overnight.
        3. Top with mixed berries before serving.

4. **Whole Grain Avocado Toast**

- **Ingredients:**
  - 2 slices whole grain bread
  - 1 avocado
  - Salt and pepper to taste
  - 1 tablespoon chia seeds
  - 1/4 cup cherry tomatoes, halved
- **Instructions:**
  1. Toast the whole grain bread.
  2. Mash the avocado and spread it on the toast.
  3. Sprinkle with salt, pepper, and chia seeds.
  4. Top with cherry tomatoes.

5. **Quinoa Breakfast Bowl**

- **Ingredients:**
  - 1/2 cup cooked quinoa
  - 1/2 cup Greek yogurt
  - 1/4 cup mixed berries
  - 1 tablespoon honey
  - 1 tablespoon flax seeds
- **Instructions:**
  1. Combine the cooked quinoa and Greek yogurt in a bowl.
  2. Top with mixed berries, honey, and flax seeds.

6. **High-Fiber Pancakes with Berries**

- **Ingredients:**
  - 1 cup whole wheat flour
  - 1 tablespoon baking powder
  - 1 tablespoon flaxseed meal
  - 1 cup almond milk
  - 1 egg
  - 1 teaspoon vanilla extract
  - 1/2 cup mixed berries

- Maple syrup for serving
- **Instructions:**
    1. Mix the whole wheat flour, baking powder, and flaxseed meal in a bowl.
    2. In another bowl, whisk the almond milk, egg, and vanilla extract.
    3. Combine the wet and dry ingredients until smooth.
    4. Fold in the mixed berries.
    5. Cook on a non-stick griddle over medium heat until bubbles form on the surface, then flip and cook until golden brown.
    6. Serve with maple syrup.

7. **Spinach and Mushroom Omelet**

    - **Ingredients:**
        - 2 eggs
        - 1/2 cup spinach
        - 1/4 cup sliced mushrooms
        - Salt and pepper to taste
        - 1 tablespoon olive oil
    - **Instructions:**
        1. Whisk the eggs in a bowl.
        2. Heat the olive oil in a pan and sauté the spinach and mushrooms until soft.
        3. Pour the eggs over the vegetables and cook until set.
        4. Season with salt and pepper.

8. **Almond Butter and Banana Smoothie**

    - **Ingredients:**
        - 1 banana
        - 1 tablespoon almond butter
        - 1 cup almond milk
        - 1 tablespoon chia seeds

- 1 teaspoon honey
- **Instructions:**
    1. Blend all ingredients until smooth.
    2. Serve immediately.

9. **High-Fiber Muffins**

    - **Ingredients:**
        - 1 cup whole wheat flour
        - 1/2 cup oat bran
        - 1/2 cup applesauce
        - 1/4 cup honey
        - 1/2 cup almond milk
        - 1 egg
        - 1 teaspoon baking powder
        - 1/2 cup mixed berries
    - **Instructions:**
        1. Preheat oven to 350°F (175°C).
        2. Mix the whole wheat flour, oat bran, and baking powder in a bowl.
        3. In another bowl, combine the applesauce, honey, almond milk, and egg.
        4. Mix the wet and dry ingredients until just combined.
        5. Fold in the mixed berries.
        6. Divide the batter into a muffin tin and bake for 20-25 minutes.

10. **Mixed Berry Parfait**

    - **Ingredients:**
        - 1 cup Greek yogurt
        - 1/2 cup mixed berries
        - 1/4 cup granola
        - 1 tablespoon honey
    - **Instructions:**

1. Layer the Greek yogurt, mixed berries, and granola in a glass.
2. Drizzle with honey before serving.

Lunch Recipes

1. **Quinoa Salad with Vegetables and Feta**

    - **Ingredients:**
        - 1 cup cooked quinoa
        - 1/2 cup cherry tomatoes, halved
        - 1/2 cup cucumber, diced
        - 1/4 cup red onion, diced
        - 1/4 cup feta cheese, crumbled
        - 2 tablespoons olive oil
        - 1 tablespoon lemon juice
        - Salt and pepper to taste
    - **Instructions:**
        1. Combine the quinoa, cherry tomatoes, cucumber, red onion, and feta cheese in a bowl.
        2. Drizzle with olive oil and lemon juice.
        3. Season with salt and pepper.
2. **Lentil Soup**

    - **Ingredients:**
        - 1 cup lentils, rinsed
        - 1 onion, chopped
        - 2 carrots, chopped
        - 2 celery stalks, chopped
        - 3 garlic cloves, minced
        - 1 can (14.5 oz) diced tomatoes
        - 4 cups vegetable broth
        - 1 tablespoon olive oil

- 1 teaspoon cumin
- 1 teaspoon paprika
- Salt and pepper to taste

- **Instructions:**
    1. Heat olive oil in a pot and sauté the onion, carrots, celery, and garlic until softened.
    2. Add the lentils, diced tomatoes, vegetable broth, cumin, and paprika.
    3. Bring to a boil, then reduce heat and simmer for 30-40 minutes, or until lentils are tender.
    4. Season with salt and pepper.

3. **Chickpea and Avocado Salad**

    - **Ingredients:**
        - 1 can (15 oz) chickpeas, drained and rinsed
        - 1 avocado, diced
        - 1/2 cup cherry tomatoes, halved
        - 1/4 cup red onion, diced
        - 2 tablespoons olive oil
        - 1 tablespoon lemon juice
        - Salt and pepper to taste
    - **Instructions:**
        1. Combine the chickpeas, avocado, cherry tomatoes, and red onion in a bowl.
        2. Drizzle with olive oil and lemon juice.
        3. Season with salt and pepper.

4. **Veggie Wrap with Hummus**

    - **Ingredients:**
        - 1 whole grain wrap
        - 1/4 cup hummus
        - 1/2 cup mixed greens
        - 1/4 cup shredded carrots

- 1/4 cup sliced cucumber
- 1/4 cup red bell pepper, sliced
◦ **Instructions:**
  1. Spread the hummus on the wrap.
  2. Layer the mixed greens, shredded carrots, cucumber, and red bell pepper on top.
  3. Roll up the wrap and slice in half.

5. **Black Bean and Corn Salad**

   ◦ **Ingredients:**
     - 1 can (15 oz) black beans, drained and rinsed
     - 1 cup corn kernels
     - 1/2 cup cherry tomatoes, halved
     - 1/4 cup red onion, diced
     - 1/4 cup cilantro, chopped
     - 2 tablespoons olive oil
     - 1 tablespoon lime juice
     - Salt and pepper to taste
   ◦ **Instructions:**
     1. Combine the black beans, corn, cherry tomatoes, red onion, and cilantro in a bowl.
     2. Drizzle with olive oil and lime juice.
     3. Season with salt and pepper.

6. **Roasted Veggie and Farro Bowl**

   ◦ **Ingredients:**
     - 1 cup cooked farro
     - 1 cup mixed roasted vegetables (zucchini, bell peppers, carrots)
     - 1/4 cup feta cheese, crumbled
     - 2 tablespoons olive oil
     - 1 tablespoon balsamic vinegar
     - Salt and pepper to taste

- **Instructions:**
    1. Combine the cooked farro, roasted vegetables, and feta cheese in a bowl.
    2. Drizzle with olive oil and balsamic vinegar.
    3. Season with salt and pepper.
7. **Sweet Potato and Black Bean Chili**

    - **Ingredients:**
        - 1 large sweet potato, peeled and diced
        - 1 can (15 oz) black beans, drained and rinsed
        - 1 can (14.5 oz) diced tomatoes
        - 1 onion, chopped
        - 2 garlic cloves, minced
        - 1 tablespoon olive oil
        - 1 teaspoon cumin
        - 1 teaspoon chili powder
        - 2 cups vegetable broth
        - Salt and pepper to taste
    - **Instructions:**
        1. Heat olive oil in a pot and sauté the onion and garlic until softened.
        2. Add the diced sweet potato, black beans, diced tomatoes, vegetable broth, cumin, and chili powder.
        3. Bring to a boil, then reduce heat and simmer for 25-30 minutes, or until sweet potatoes are tender.
        4. Season with salt and pepper.
8. **Spinach and Strawberry Salad**

    - **Ingredients:**
        - 2 cups fresh spinach
        - 1 cup sliced strawberries
        - 1/4 cup sliced almonds
        - 1/4 cup feta cheese, crumbled

- 2 tablespoons balsamic vinaigrette
- Instructions:
    1. Combine the spinach, strawberries, sliced almonds, and feta cheese in a bowl.
    2. Drizzle with balsamic vinaigrette before serving.

9. **Mediterranean Grain Bowl**

    - Ingredients:
        - 1 cup cooked farro
        - 1/2 cup cherry tomatoes, halved
        - 1/2 cup cucumber, diced
        - 1/4 cup kalamata olives, sliced
        - 1/4 cup feta cheese, crumbled
        - 2 tablespoons olive oil
        - 1 tablespoon lemon juice
        - Salt and pepper to taste
    - Instructions:
        1. Combine the cooked farro, cherry tomatoes, cucumber, kalamata olives, and feta cheese in a bowl.
        2. Drizzle with olive oil and lemon juice.
        3. Season with salt and pepper.

10. **Tabbouleh with Fresh Herbs**

    - Ingredients:
        - 1 cup cooked bulgur wheat
        - 1/2 cup chopped parsley
        - 1/4 cup chopped mint
        - 1/2 cup cherry tomatoes, diced
        - 1/4 cup cucumber, diced
        - 2 tablespoons olive oil
        - 1 tablespoon lemon juice
        - Salt and pepper to taste
    - Instructions:

1. Combine the cooked bulgur wheat, parsley, mint, cherry tomatoes, and cucumber in a bowl.
2. Drizzle with olive oil and lemon juice.
3. Season with salt and pepper.

Dinner Recipes

1. **Baked Salmon with Quinoa and Steamed Veggies**

   - **Ingredients:**
     - 2 salmon fillets
     - 1 cup cooked quinoa
     - 1 cup steamed broccoli
     - 1 cup steamed carrots
     - 2 tablespoons olive oil
     - 1 tablespoon lemon juice
     - Salt and pepper to taste
   - **Instructions:**
     1. Preheat oven to 375°F (190°C).
     2. Place the salmon fillets on a baking sheet, drizzle with olive oil and lemon juice, and season with salt and pepper.
     3. Bake for 15-20 minutes, or until the salmon is cooked through.
     4. Serve with cooked quinoa, steamed broccoli, and steamed carrots.

2. **Stuffed Bell Peppers with Brown Rice**

   - **Ingredients:**
     - 4 bell peppers, tops cut off and seeds removed
     - 1 cup cooked brown rice
     - 1/2 cup black beans, drained and rinsed
     - 1/2 cup corn kernels

- 1/2 cup diced tomatoes
- 1/4 cup diced onion
- 1 tablespoon olive oil
- 1 teaspoon cumin
- 1 teaspoon chili powder
- Salt and pepper to taste

◦ **Instructions**:
1. Preheat oven to 375°F (190°C).
2. Heat olive oil in a pan and sauté the onion until softened.
3. Add the black beans, corn, diced tomatoes, cooked brown rice, cumin, and chili powder. Season with salt and pepper.
4. Stuff the bell peppers with the rice mixture and place in a baking dish.
5. Bake for 30-35 minutes, or until the bell peppers are tender.

3. **Spaghetti Squash with Marinara Sauce**

    ◦ **Ingredients**:
    - 1 spaghetti squash
    - 2 cups marinara sauce
    - 1/4 cup grated Parmesan cheese
    - 1 tablespoon olive oil
    - Salt and pepper to taste

    ◦ **Instructions**:
    1. Preheat oven to 400°F (200°C).
    2. Cut the spaghetti squash in half lengthwise and remove the seeds.
    3. Drizzle with olive oil and season with salt and pepper.
    4. Place the squash halves cut side down on a baking sheet and bake for 40-45 minutes, or until tender.

5. Use a fork to scrape out the strands of squash and serve with marinara sauce and grated Parmesan cheese.

4. **Grilled Chicken with Barley and Roasted Vegetables**

   - **Ingredients:**
     - 2 chicken breasts
     - 1 cup cooked barley
     - 1 cup roasted vegetables (zucchini, bell peppers, carrots)
     - 2 tablespoons olive oil
     - 1 tablespoon balsamic vinegar
     - Salt and pepper to taste
   - **Instructions:**
     1. Preheat grill to medium-high heat.
     2. Season the chicken breasts with olive oil, balsamic vinegar, salt, and pepper.
     3. Grill the chicken for 6-7 minutes per side, or until fully cooked.
     4. Serve with cooked barley and roasted vegetables.

5. **Eggplant Parmesan**

   - **Ingredients:**
     - 1 large eggplant, sliced into rounds
     - 2 cups marinara sauce
     - 1 cup shredded mozzarella cheese
     - 1/4 cup grated Parmesan cheese
     - 1 cup whole wheat breadcrumbs
     - 2 eggs, beaten
     - 1 tablespoon olive oil
     - Salt and pepper to taste
   - **Instructions:**
     1. Preheat oven to 375°F (190°C).

2. Dip the eggplant slices in beaten egg, then coat with whole wheat breadcrumbs.
3. Heat olive oil in a pan and cook the eggplant slices until golden brown on both sides.
4. In a baking dish, layer the eggplant slices, marinara sauce, and shredded mozzarella cheese.
5. Sprinkle with grated Parmesan cheese and bake for 20-25 minutes, or until the cheese is melted and bubbly.

6. **High-Fiber Veggie Stir-Fry**

    - **Ingredients:**
        - 1 cup broccoli florets
        - 1 cup sliced bell peppers
        - 1 cup snap peas
        - 1 cup sliced carrots
        - 1 cup cooked brown rice
        - 2 tablespoons soy sauce
        - 1 tablespoon olive oil
        - 1 tablespoon sesame seeds
        - 2 garlic cloves, minced
        - Salt and pepper to taste
    - **Instructions:**
    1. Heat olive oil in a large pan and sauté the garlic until fragrant.
    2. Add the broccoli, bell peppers, snap peas, and carrots. Stir-fry until vegetables are tender-crisp.
    3. Stir in the cooked brown rice and soy sauce. Cook for another 2-3 minutes.
    4. Sprinkle with sesame seeds before serving.

7. **Quinoa and Black Bean Stuffed Sweet Potatoes**

    - **Ingredients:**

- 4 medium sweet potatoes
- 1 cup cooked quinoa
- 1 can (15 oz) black beans, drained and rinsed
- 1/2 cup corn kernels
- 1/4 cup diced red onion
- 2 tablespoons olive oil
- 1 tablespoon lime juice
- 1 teaspoon cumin
- 1 teaspoon chili powder
- Salt and pepper to taste

◦ **Instructions:**
  1. Preheat oven to 400°F (200°C).
  2. Prick the sweet potatoes with a fork and bake for 45-50 minutes, or until tender.
  3. In a pan, heat olive oil and sauté the red onion until softened.
  4. Add the black beans, corn, cooked quinoa, cumin, and chili powder. Season with salt and pepper.
  5. Cut the sweet potatoes in half and scoop out a small portion of the flesh.
  6. Fill the sweet potatoes with the quinoa mixture and drizzle with lime juice.

8. **Turkey and Vegetable Meatloaf**

◦ **Ingredients:**
  - 1 pound ground turkey
  - 1/2 cup finely chopped carrots
  - 1/2 cup finely chopped celery
  - 1/2 cup finely chopped onion
  - 1/4 cup whole wheat breadcrumbs
  - 1 egg, beaten
  - 2 tablespoons ketchup
  - 1 tablespoon Worcestershire sauce

- 1 tablespoon olive oil
- Salt and pepper to taste

- **Instructions**:
  1. Preheat oven to 375°F (190°C).
  2. In a pan, heat olive oil and sauté the carrots, celery, and onion until softened.
  3. In a bowl, combine the ground turkey, sautéed vegetables, whole wheat breadcrumbs, beaten egg, ketchup, Worcestershire sauce, salt, and pepper.
  4. Form the mixture into a loaf shape and place in a baking dish.
  5. Bake for 45-50 minutes, or until the meatloaf is fully cooked.

9. **Whole Wheat Pasta Primavera**

    - **Ingredients**:
      - 8 ounces whole wheat pasta
      - 1 cup broccoli florets
      - 1 cup sliced bell peppers
      - 1 cup cherry tomatoes, halved
      - 1/2 cup sliced zucchini
      - 2 garlic cloves, minced
      - 2 tablespoons olive oil
      - 1/4 cup grated Parmesan cheese
      - Salt and pepper to taste
    - **Instructions**:
      1. Cook the whole wheat pasta according to package instructions.
      2. In a large pan, heat olive oil and sauté the garlic until fragrant.
      3. Add the broccoli, bell peppers, cherry tomatoes, and zucchini. Cook until the vegetables are tender.

4. Drain the pasta and add it to the pan with the vegetables.
   5. Toss to combine and season with salt and pepper.
   6. Sprinkle with grated Parmesan cheese before serving.

10. **Red Lentil Curry**

   - **Ingredients:**
     - 1 cup red lentils, rinsed
     - 1 onion, chopped
     - 2 garlic cloves, minced
     - 1 tablespoon grated ginger
     - 1 can (14.5 oz) diced tomatoes
     - 1 can (13.5 oz) coconut milk
     - 2 cups vegetable broth
     - 1 tablespoon curry powder
     - 1 teaspoon cumin
     - 1 teaspoon turmeric
     - 1 tablespoon olive oil
     - Salt and pepper to taste
   - **Instructions:**
     1. Heat olive oil in a pot and sauté the onion, garlic, and grated ginger until softened.
     2. Add the curry powder, cumin, and turmeric. Cook for another 1-2 minutes.
     3. Stir in the diced tomatoes, coconut milk, vegetable broth, and red lentils.
     4. Bring to a boil, then reduce heat and simmer for 25-30 minutes, or until the lentils are tender.
     5. Season with salt and pepper before serving.

Snacks and Desserts

1. **Chia Seed Pudding**

- **Ingredients:**
  - 1/4 cup chia seeds
  - 1 cup almond milk
  - 1 tablespoon honey
  - 1/2 cup mixed berries
- **Instructions:**
  1. Mix the chia seeds, almond milk, and honey in a bowl.
  2. Refrigerate for at least 4 hours or overnight.
  3. Top with mixed berries before serving.

2. **Baked Apple Slices with Cinnamon**

   - **Ingredients:**
     - 2 apples, sliced
     - 1 tablespoon cinnamon
     - 1 tablespoon honey
   - **Instructions:**
     1. Preheat oven to 350°F (175°C).
     2. Arrange the apple slices on a baking sheet.
     3. Sprinkle with cinnamon and drizzle with honey.
     4. Bake for 20-25 minutes, or until the apples are tender.

3. **High-Fiber Energy Bars**

   - **Ingredients:**
     - 1 cup rolled oats
     - 1/2 cup almond butter
     - 1/4 cup honey
     - 1/4 cup chia seeds
     - 1/4 cup flaxseed meal
     - 1/4 cup dried cranberries
   - **Instructions:**
     1. Mix all ingredients in a bowl until well combined.

2. Press the mixture into a lined baking dish.
3. Refrigerate for at least 1 hour, then cut into bars.

4. **Hummus with Veggie Sticks**

   - **Ingredients:**
     - 1 can (15 oz) chickpeas, drained and rinsed
     - 1/4 cup tahini
     - 2 tablespoons olive oil
     - 1 garlic clove, minced
     - 1 tablespoon lemon juice
     - 1/4 cup water
     - Salt and pepper to taste
     - Assorted veggie sticks (carrots, celery, bell peppers)
   - **Instructions:**
     1. Blend the chickpeas, tahini, olive oil, garlic, lemon juice, and water until smooth.
     2. Season with salt and pepper.
     3. Serve with assorted veggie sticks.

5. **Fruit and Nut Trail Mix**

   - **Ingredients:**
     - 1/2 cup almonds
     - 1/2 cup walnuts
     - 1/2 cup dried cranberries
     - 1/2 cup raisins
     - 1/2 cup sunflower seeds
   - **Instructions:**
     1. Mix all ingredients in a bowl.
     2. Store in an airtight container.

6. **Almond Flour Cookies**

   - **Ingredients:**
     - 1 cup almond flour

- 1/4 cup honey
- 1/4 cup coconut oil, melted
- 1 teaspoon vanilla extract
- 1/4 teaspoon baking soda
- Pinch of salt

◦ **Instructions:**
1. Preheat oven to 350°F (175°C).
2. Mix all ingredients in a bowl until well combined.
3. Drop spoonfuls of dough onto a lined baking sheet.
4. Bake for 10-12 minutes, or until golden brown.

7. **Berry Smoothie**

    ◦ **Ingredients:**
    - 1 cup mixed berries
    - 1 banana
    - 1 cup almond milk
    - 1 tablespoon chia seeds
    - 1 teaspoon honey

    ◦ **Instructions:**
    1. Blend all ingredients until smooth.
    2. Serve immediately.

8. **Greek Yogurt with Honey and Nuts**

    ◦ **Ingredients:**
    - 1 cup Greek yogurt
    - 1 tablespoon honey
    - 1/4 cup mixed nuts (almonds, walnuts)

    ◦ **Instructions:**
    1. Top the Greek yogurt with honey and mixed nuts.
    2. Serve immediately.

9. **Baked Pears with Walnuts**

    ◦ **Ingredients:**

- 2 pears, halved and cored
- 1/4 cup chopped walnuts
- 1 tablespoon honey
- 1/2 teaspoon cinnamon

◦ **Instructions:**
1. Preheat oven to 350°F (175°C).
2. Place the pear halves in a baking dish.
3. Top with chopped walnuts, honey, and cinnamon.
4. Bake for 20-25 minutes, or until the pears are tender.

10. **High-Fiber Banana Bread**

◦ **Ingredients:**
- 2 cups whole wheat flour
- 1 teaspoon baking soda
- 1/2 teaspoon salt
- 1/2 cup unsweetened applesauce
- 1/4 cup honey
- 2 eggs
- 3 ripe bananas, mashed
- 1 teaspoon vanilla extract

◦ **Instructions:**
1. Preheat oven to 350°F (175°C).
2. Mix the whole wheat flour, baking soda, and salt in a bowl.
3. In another bowl, combine the applesauce, honey, eggs, mashed bananas, and vanilla extract.
4. Mix the wet and dry ingredients until just combined.
5. Pour the batter into a greased loaf pan and bake for 50-60 minutes, or until a toothpick inserted into the center comes out clean.

11. **Quinoa Salad with Vegetables and Feta**

◦ **Ingredients:**

- 1 cup cooked quinoa
- 1/2 cup cherry tomatoes, halved
- 1/2 cup cucumber, diced
- 1/4 cup red onion, diced
- 1/4 cup feta cheese, crumbled
- 2 tablespoons olive oil
- 1 tablespoon lemon juice
- Salt and pepper to taste

- **Instructions:**
    1. Combine the quinoa, cherry tomatoes, cucumber, red onion, and feta cheese in a bowl.
    2. Drizzle with olive oil and lemon juice.
    3. Season with salt and pepper.

12. **Lentil Soup**

    - **Ingredients:**
        - 1 cup lentils, rinsed
        - 1 onion, chopped
        - 2 carrots, chopped
        - 2 celery stalks, chopped
        - 3 garlic cloves, minced
        - 1 can (14.5 oz) diced tomatoes
        - 4 cups vegetable broth
        - 1 tablespoon olive oil
        - 1 teaspoon cumin
        - 1 teaspoon paprika
        - Salt and pepper to taste
    - **Instructions:**
        1. Heat olive oil in a pot and sauté the onion, carrots, celery, and garlic until softened.
        2. Add the lentils, diced tomatoes, vegetable broth, cumin, and paprika.

3. Bring to a boil, then reduce heat and simmer for 30-40 minutes, or until lentils are tender.
4. Season with salt and pepper.

13. **Chickpea and Avocado Salad**

    - **Ingredients:**
        - 1 can (15 oz) chickpeas, drained and rinsed
        - 1 avocado, diced
        - 1/2 cup cherry tomatoes, halved
        - 1/4 cup red onion, diced
        - 2 tablespoons olive oil
        - 1 tablespoon lemon juice
        - Salt and pepper to taste
    - **Instructions:**
        1. Combine the chickpeas, avocado, cherry tomatoes, and red onion in a bowl.
        2. Drizzle with olive oil and lemon juice.
        3. Season with salt and pepper.

14. **Veggie Wrap with Hummus**

    - **Ingredients:**
        - 1 whole grain wrap
        - 1/4 cup hummus
        - 1/2 cup mixed greens
        - 1/4 cup shredded carrots
        - 1/4 cup sliced cucumber
        - 1/4 cup red bell pepper, sliced
    - **Instructions:**
        1. Spread the hummus on the wrap.
        2. Layer the mixed greens, shredded carrots, cucumber, and red bell pepper on top.
        3. Roll up the wrap and slice in half.

15. **Black Bean and Corn Salad**

- Ingredients:
  - 1 can (15 oz) black beans, drained and rinsed
  - 1 cup corn kernels
  - 1/2 cup cherry tomatoes, halved
  - 1/4 cup red onion, diced
  - 1/4 cup cilantro, chopped
  - 2 tablespoons olive oil
  - 1 tablespoon lime juice
  - Salt and pepper to taste
- Instructions:
  1. Combine the black beans, corn, cherry tomatoes, red onion, and cilantro in a bowl.
  2. Drizzle with olive oil and lime juice.
  3. Season with salt and pepper.

16. **Roasted Veggie and Farro Bowl**

- Ingredients:
  - 1 cup cooked farro
  - 1 cup mixed roasted vegetables (zucchini, bell peppers, carrots)
  - 1/4 cup feta cheese, crumbled
  - 2 tablespoons olive oil
  - 1 tablespoon balsamic vinegar
  - Salt and pepper to taste
- Instructions:
  1. Combine the cooked farro, roasted vegetables, and feta cheese in a bowl.
  2. Drizzle with olive oil and balsamic vinegar.
  3. Season with salt and pepper.

17. **Sweet Potato and Black Bean Chili**

- Ingredients:
  - 1 large sweet potato, peeled and diced

- 1 can (15 oz) black beans, drained and rinsed
- 1 can (14.5 oz) diced tomatoes
- 1 onion, chopped
- 2 garlic cloves, minced
- 1 tablespoon olive oil
- 1 teaspoon cumin
- 1 teaspoon chili powder
- 2 cups vegetable broth
- Salt and pepper to taste

◦ **Instructions:**
1. Heat olive oil in a pot and sauté the onion and garlic until softened.
2. Add the diced sweet potato, black beans, diced tomatoes, vegetable broth, cumin, and chili powder.
3. Bring to a boil, then reduce heat and simmer for 25-30 minutes, or until sweet potatoes are tender.
4. Season with salt and pepper.

18. **Spinach and Strawberry Salad**

◦ **Ingredients:**
- 2 cups fresh spinach
- 1 cup sliced strawberries
- 1/4 cup sliced almonds
- 1/4 cup feta cheese, crumbled
- 2 tablespoons balsamic vinaigrette

◦ **Instructions:**
1. Combine the spinach, strawberries, sliced almonds, and feta cheese in a bowl.
2. Drizzle with balsamic vinaigrette before serving.

19. **Mediterranean Grain Bowl**

◦ **Ingredients:**
- 1 cup cooked farro

- 1/2 cup cherry tomatoes, halved
- 1/2 cup cucumber, diced
- 1/4 cup kalamata olives, sliced
- 1/4 cup feta cheese, crumbled
- 2 tablespoons olive oil
- 1 tablespoon lemon juice
- Salt and pepper to taste

- **Instructions:**
  1. Combine the cooked farro, cherry tomatoes, cucumber, kalamata olives, and feta cheese in a bowl.
  2. Drizzle with olive oil and lemon juice.
  3. Season with salt and pepper.

20. **Tabbouleh with Fresh Herbs**

- **Ingredients:**
  - 1 cup cooked bulgur wheat
  - 1/2 cup chopped parsley
  - 1/4 cup chopped mint
  - 1/2 cup cherry tomatoes, diced
  - 1/4 cup cucumber, diced
  - 2 tablespoons olive oil
  - 1 tablespoon lemon juice
  - Salt and pepper to taste

- **Instructions:**
  1. Combine the cooked bulgur wheat, parsley, mint, cherry tomatoes, and cucumber in a bowl.
  2. Drizzle with olive oil and lemon juice.
  3. Season with salt and pepper.

4

Low-Residue Recipes for Flare-Up Periods

During flare-up periods, it's essential to follow a low-residue diet to minimize irritation and allow your digestive system to heal. Here are 35 soothing and gentle low-residue recipes.

Breakfast Recipes

1. **Smooth Banana Oatmeal**

    - **Ingredients**:
        - 1/2 cup quick oats
        - 1 cup water or milk
        - 1 ripe banana, mashed
        - 1 teaspoon honey
    - **Instructions**:
        1. Bring the water or milk to a boil in a pot.
        2. Add the quick oats and reduce the heat to a simmer. Cook for about 3-5 minutes, stirring occasionally.
        3. Stir in the mashed banana and honey. Serve warm.
2. **Scrambled Eggs with White Toast**

- Ingredients:
    - 2 eggs
    - 2 tablespoons milk
    - 1 tablespoon butter
    - Salt and pepper to taste
    - 2 slices white bread, toasted
- Instructions:
    1. Whisk the eggs and milk in a bowl.
    2. Melt the butter in a pan over medium heat.
    3. Pour in the eggs and cook, stirring gently, until set.
    4. Season with salt and pepper and serve with white toast.

3. **Rice Porridge**

    - Ingredients:
        - 1/2 cup white rice
        - 2 cups water or chicken broth
        - Salt to taste
    - Instructions:
        1. Rinse the rice and place it in a pot with water or chicken broth.
        2. Bring to a boil, then reduce heat and simmer for 30-40 minutes, stirring occasionally, until the rice is very soft and the mixture is thick.
        3. Season with salt to taste and serve warm.

4. **Smooth Applesauce Pancakes**

    - Ingredients:
        - 1 cup white flour
        - 1 tablespoon sugar
        - 1 teaspoon baking powder
        - 1/2 teaspoon baking soda
        - 1 cup buttermilk

- 1/2 cup applesauce
- 1 egg
- 2 tablespoons butter, melted

○ **Instructions**:
1. Mix the white flour, sugar, baking powder, and baking soda in a bowl.
2. In another bowl, combine the buttermilk, applesauce, egg, and melted butter.
3. Combine the wet and dry ingredients until just blended.
4. Cook on a non-stick griddle over medium heat until bubbles form on the surface, then flip and cook until golden brown. Serve warm.

5. **White Bread French Toast**

   ○ **Ingredients**:
   - 2 slices white bread
   - 1 egg
   - 1/4 cup milk
   - 1 teaspoon vanilla extract
   - 1/2 teaspoon cinnamon
   - 1 tablespoon butter
   - Maple syrup for serving

   ○ **Instructions**:
   1. Whisk the egg, milk, vanilla extract, and cinnamon in a bowl.
   2. Dip the bread slices into the mixture, coating both sides.
   3. Melt the butter in a pan over medium heat and cook the bread slices until golden brown on both sides.
   4. Serve with maple syrup.

6. **Rice Flour Muffins**

- **Ingredients:**
  - 1 cup rice flour
  - 1/4 cup sugar
  - 1 teaspoon baking powder
  - 1/2 teaspoon salt
  - 1/2 cup milk
  - 1/4 cup vegetable oil
  - 1 egg
- **Instructions:**
  1. Preheat oven to 350°F (175°C).
  2. Mix the rice flour, sugar, baking powder, and salt in a bowl.
  3. In another bowl, combine the milk, vegetable oil, and egg.
  4. Mix the wet and dry ingredients until just combined.
  5. Pour the batter into a greased muffin tin and bake for 15-20 minutes.

7. **Soft-Boiled Eggs with Toast**

   - **Ingredients:**
     - 2 eggs
     - 2 slices white bread, toasted
   - **Instructions:**
     1. Bring a pot of water to a boil.
     2. Gently place the eggs in the boiling water and cook for 6-7 minutes.
     3. Remove the eggs and place them in cold water to cool slightly.
     4. Peel the eggs and serve with toasted white bread.

8. **Low-Residue Smoothie**

   - **Ingredients:**
     - 1 banana

- 1/2 cup plain yogurt
- 1/2 cup almond milk
- 1 tablespoon honey

◦ **Instructions:**
1. Blend all ingredients until smooth.
2. Serve immediately.

Lunch Recipes

1. **Chicken and Rice Soup**

    ◦ **Ingredients:**
    - 1 chicken breast, cooked and shredded
    - 1/2 cup white rice
    - 1 carrot, finely diced
    - 1 celery stalk, finely diced
    - 1/2 onion, finely diced
    - 4 cups chicken broth
    - Salt and pepper to taste

    ◦ **Instructions:**
    1. In a pot, combine the chicken broth, carrot, celery, and onion. Bring to a boil.
    2. Add the white rice and reduce heat to a simmer. Cook for about 20 minutes, or until the rice is tender.
    3. Stir in the cooked chicken and season with salt and pepper.

2. **Mashed Potatoes with Grilled Chicken**

    ◦ **Ingredients:**
    - 2 medium potatoes, peeled and diced
    - 1 chicken breast
    - 2 tablespoons butter
    - 1/4 cup milk

- Salt and pepper to taste
- **Instructions:**
  1. Boil the potatoes in salted water until tender, about 15 minutes.
  2. Drain and mash the potatoes with butter and milk. Season with salt and pepper.
  3. Season the chicken breast with salt and pepper and grill until fully cooked.
  4. Serve the mashed potatoes with the grilled chicken.

3. **White Rice and Steamed Fish**

   - **Ingredients:**
     - 1 cup white rice
     - 2 white fish fillets
     - 1 tablespoon olive oil
     - Salt and pepper to taste
   - **Instructions:**
     1. Cook the white rice according to package instructions.
     2. Season the fish fillets with salt and pepper.
     3. Steam the fish fillets until fully cooked.
     4. Serve the steamed fish with the white rice.

4. **Carrot and Potato Puree**

   - **Ingredients:**
     - 2 medium potatoes, peeled and diced
     - 2 carrots, peeled and diced
     - 1 tablespoon butter
     - 1/4 cup milk
     - Salt and pepper to taste
   - **Instructions:**
     1. Boil the potatoes and carrots in salted water until tender, about 15 minutes.

2. Drain and mash the potatoes and carrots with butter and milk. Season with salt and pepper.

5. **Smooth Tomato Soup**

    - Ingredients:
        - 4 cups tomatoes, peeled and chopped
        - 1 onion, chopped
        - 2 garlic cloves, minced
        - 2 cups chicken broth
        - 1 tablespoon olive oil
        - Salt and pepper to taste
    - Instructions:
        1. Heat olive oil in a pot and sauté the onion and garlic until softened.
        2. Add the tomatoes and chicken broth. Bring to a boil, then reduce heat and simmer for 20-25 minutes.
        3. Blend the soup until smooth and season with salt and pepper.

6. **Soft White Bread Sandwich with Turkey**

    - Ingredients:
        - 2 slices white bread
        - 3 slices deli turkey
        - 1 tablespoon mayonnaise
        - Salt and pepper to taste
    - Instructions:
        1. Spread the mayonnaise on the white bread slices.
        2. Layer the deli turkey on one slice of bread.
        3. Season with salt and pepper and top with the other slice of bread.

7. **Rice and Egg Salad**

    - Ingredients:

- 1 cup cooked white rice
- 2 hard-boiled eggs, chopped
- 1/4 cup mayonnaise
- 1 tablespoon lemon juice
- Salt and pepper to taste

◦ **Instructions**:
1. Combine the cooked white rice, chopped eggs, mayonnaise, and lemon juice in a bowl.
2. Season with salt and pepper.

8. **Mild Chicken Curry with White Rice**

   ◦ **Ingredients**:
   - 1 chicken breast, cubed
   - 1 cup white rice
   - 1 onion, finely chopped
   - 1 garlic clove, minced
   - 1 tablespoon curry powder
   - 1 cup coconut milk
   - 1 tablespoon olive oil
   - Salt and pepper to taste

   ◦ **Instructions**:
   1. Cook the white rice according to package instructions.
   2. Heat olive oil in a pot and sauté the onion and garlic until softened.
   3. Add the cubed chicken and cook until no longer pink.
   4. Stir in the curry powder and coconut milk. Simmer for 10-15 minutes.
   5. Season with salt and pepper and serve with the white rice.

9. **Smooth Vegetable Soup**

- **Ingredients:**
    - 2 cups mixed vegetables (carrots, potatoes, zucchini), peeled and chopped
    - 1 onion, chopped
    - 2 garlic cloves, minced
    - 4 cups vegetable broth
    - 1 tablespoon olive oil
    - Salt and pepper to taste
- **Instructions:**
    1. Heat olive oil in a pot and sauté the onion and garlic until softened.
    2. Add the mixed vegetables and vegetable broth. Bring to a boil, then reduce heat and simmer for 20-25 minutes.
    3. Blend the soup until smooth and season with salt and pepper.

Dinner Recipes

1. **Baked Cod with Carrot Puree**

    - **Ingredients:**
        - 2 cod fillets
        - 4 carrots, peeled and diced
        - 1 tablespoon olive oil
        - 1/4 cup milk
        - Salt and pepper to taste
    - **Instructions:**
        1. Preheat oven to 375°F (190°C).
        2. Season the cod fillets with salt and pepper and drizzle with olive oil.
        3. Bake the cod for 15-20 minutes, or until fully cooked.

4. Boil the carrots in salted water until tender, about 15 minutes.
   5. Drain and puree the carrots with milk. Season with salt and pepper.
   6. Serve the baked cod with carrot puree.

2. **Pasta with Butter and Parmesan**

   - **Ingredients**:
     - 8 ounces white pasta
     - 1/4 cup butter
     - 1/4 cup grated Parmesan cheese
     - Salt and pepper to taste
   - **Instructions**:
     1. Cook the pasta according to package instructions.
     2. Drain the pasta and return it to the pot.
     3. Stir in the butter until melted.
     4. Add the grated Parmesan cheese and season with salt and pepper. Serve warm.

3. **Rice and Ground Turkey Casserole**

   - **Ingredients**:
     - 1 pound ground turkey
     - 1 cup cooked white rice
     - 1 onion, finely chopped
     - 1 garlic clove, minced
     - 1 cup chicken broth
     - 1 tablespoon olive oil
     - Salt and pepper to taste
   - **Instructions**:
     1. Preheat oven to 350°F (175°C).
     2. Heat olive oil in a pan and sauté the onion and garlic until softened.

3. Add the ground turkey and cook until no longer pink. Season with salt and pepper.
4. In a baking dish, combine the cooked white rice, ground turkey, and chicken broth.
5. Bake for 20-25 minutes.

4. **Baked Chicken with Rice**

   - **Ingredients**:
     - 2 chicken breasts
     - 1 cup white rice
     - 1 cup chicken broth
     - 1 tablespoon olive oil
     - Salt and pepper to taste
   - **Instructions**:
     1. Preheat oven to 375°F (190°C).
     2. Place the chicken breasts in a baking dish and drizzle with olive oil. Season with salt and pepper.
     3. Add the white rice and chicken broth to the baking dish.
     4. Cover with foil and bake for 30-35 minutes, or until the chicken is fully cooked and the rice is tender.

5. **White Fish and Mashed Potatoes**

   - **Ingredients**:
     - 2 white fish fillets
     - 2 medium potatoes, peeled and diced
     - 1 tablespoon butter
     - 1/4 cup milk
     - Salt and pepper to taste
   - **Instructions**:
     1. Preheat oven to 375°F (190°C).
     2. Season the fish fillets with salt and pepper and place them in a baking dish.

3. Bake for 15-20 minutes, or until the fish is fully cooked.
4. Boil the potatoes in salted water until tender, about 15 minutes.
5. Drain and mash the potatoes with butter and milk. Season with salt and pepper.
6. Serve the baked fish with mashed potatoes.

6. **Soft Tofu Stir-Fry**

   - **Ingredients:**
     - 1 block soft tofu, drained and cubed
     - 1 cup mixed vegetables (carrots, zucchini, bell peppers), finely chopped
     - 1 tablespoon soy sauce
     - 1 tablespoon olive oil
     - Salt and pepper to taste
   - **Instructions:**
     1. Heat olive oil in a pan and sauté the mixed vegetables until tender.
     2. Add the cubed tofu and soy sauce.
     3. Cook for another 5-7 minutes, stirring gently.
     4. Season with salt and pepper.

7. **Simple Risotto**

   - **Ingredients:**
     - 1 cup Arborio rice
     - 1/2 onion, finely chopped
     - 2 garlic cloves, minced
     - 4 cups chicken broth
     - 1/4 cup grated Parmesan cheese
     - 1 tablespoon olive oil
     - Salt and pepper to taste
   - **Instructions:**

1. Heat olive oil in a pot and sauté the onion and garlic until softened.
   2. Add the Arborio rice and cook for 1-2 minutes, stirring constantly.
   3. Gradually add the chicken broth, one ladle at a time, stirring constantly until the liquid is absorbed before adding more.
   4. Continue this process until the rice is tender and creamy.
   5. Stir in the grated Parmesan cheese and season with salt and pepper.

8. **Mild Beef Stew with Carrots**

   - **Ingredients:**
     - 1 pound beef stew meat, cubed
     - 4 carrots, peeled and chopped
     - 1 onion, finely chopped
     - 2 garlic cloves, minced
     - 4 cups beef broth
     - 1 tablespoon olive oil
     - Salt and pepper to taste
   - **Instructions:**
     1. Heat olive oil in a pot and sauté the onion and garlic until softened.
     2. Add the beef stew meat and cook until browned on all sides.
     3. Add the chopped carrots and beef broth.
     4. Bring to a boil, then reduce heat and simmer for 1-1.5 hours, or until the beef is tender.
     5. Season with salt and pepper.

9. **Baked Chicken Breast with Smooth Veggies**

   - **Ingredients:**

- 2 chicken breasts
- 2 cups mixed vegetables (carrots, zucchini, bell peppers), peeled and chopped
- 1 tablespoon olive oil
- Salt and pepper to taste

◦ **Instructions:**
1. Preheat oven to 375°F (190°C).
2. Place the chicken breasts in a baking dish and drizzle with olive oil. Season with salt and pepper.
3. Add the mixed vegetables to the baking dish.
4. Bake for 25-30 minutes, or until the chicken is fully cooked and the vegetables are tender.

Snacks and Desserts

1. **Applesauce**

    ◦ **Ingredients:**
    - 4 apples, peeled, cored, and chopped
    - 1/2 cup water
    - 1 tablespoon honey
    - 1/2 teaspoon cinnamon

    ◦ **Instructions:**
    1. Combine the apples and water in a pot and bring to a boil.
    2. Reduce heat and simmer for 15-20 minutes, or until the apples are very soft.
    3. Mash the apples until smooth and stir in the honey and cinnamon. Serve warm or chilled.

2. **Yogurt with Honey**

    ◦ **Ingredients:**
    - 1 cup plain yogurt

- 1 tablespoon honey
- Instructions:
  1. Top the yogurt with honey before serving.

3. **Banana Pudding**

   - Ingredients:
     - 2 ripe bananas
     - 1/2 cup plain yogurt
     - 1 tablespoon honey
     - 1/2 teaspoon vanilla extract
   - Instructions:
     1. Blend the bananas, yogurt, honey, and vanilla extract until smooth.
     2. Serve immediately or refrigerate until chilled.

4. **Smooth Peanut Butter Cookies**

   - Ingredients:
     - 1 cup smooth peanut butter
     - 1/2 cup sugar
     - 1 egg
     - 1 teaspoon vanilla extract
   - Instructions:
     1. Preheat oven to 350°F (175°C).
     2. Mix all ingredients in a bowl until well combined.
     3. Drop spoonfuls of dough onto a lined baking sheet and flatten with a fork.
     4. Bake for 10-12 minutes, or until golden brown.

5. **Plain Crackers with Cheese**

   - Ingredients:
     - Plain crackers
     - Slices of mild cheese (e.g., mozzarella, cheddar)
   - Instructions:

1. Serve plain crackers with slices of mild cheese.

6. **Soft Baked Apples**

    - **Ingredients:**
        - 2 apples, cored
        - 1 tablespoon honey
        - 1/2 teaspoon cinnamon
    - **Instructions:**
        1. Preheat oven to 350°F (175°C).
        2. Place the apples in a baking dish.
        3. Drizzle with honey and sprinkle with cinnamon.
        4. Bake for 20-25 minutes, or until the apples are tender.

7. **Gelatin Dessert**

    - **Ingredients:**
        - 1 package flavored gelatin
        - 2 cups water
    - **Instructions:**
        1. Prepare the gelatin according to package instructions.
        2. Refrigerate until set.

8. **Plain Rice Cakes**

    - **Ingredients:**
        - Plain rice cakes
    - **Instructions:**
        1. Serve plain rice cakes as a simple snack.

9. **Smooth Vanilla Pudding**

    - **Ingredients:**
        - 1/2 cup sugar
        - 3 tablespoons cornstarch
        - 1/4 teaspoon salt

- 2 cups milk
- 2 teaspoons vanilla extract

◦ **Instructions:**
1. In a saucepan, combine sugar, cornstarch, and salt.
2. Gradually add milk, stirring constantly.
3. Cook over medium heat, stirring constantly, until the mixture thickens and boils.
4. Boil for 1 minute, then remove from heat.
5. Stir in vanilla extract and let cool before serving.

5

Weekly Meal Plans

Planning your meals in advance can help you stay on track with your dietary needs and ensure you're getting the right nutrients. Here are sample weekly meal plans for both high-fiber and low-residue periods, along with grocery shopping lists.

High-Fiber Weekly Meal Plan

Day 1

- **Breakfast**: High-Fiber Oatmeal with Fruits and Nuts
- **Lunch**: Quinoa Salad with Vegetables and Feta
- **Dinner**: Baked Salmon with Quinoa and Steamed Veggies
- **Snack**: Chia Seed Pudding with Berries

Day 2

- **Breakfast**: Green Smoothie Bowl
- **Lunch**: Lentil Soup
- **Dinner**: Stuffed Bell Peppers with Brown Rice
- **Snack**: Baked Apple Slices with Cinnamon

Day 3

- **Breakfast**: Whole Grain Avocado Toast
- **Lunch**: Chickpea and Avocado Salad
- **Dinner**: Spaghetti Squash with Marinara Sauce
- **Snack**: High-Fiber Energy Bars

Day 4

- **Breakfast**: Quinoa Breakfast Bowl
- **Lunch**: Veggie Wrap with Hummus
- **Dinner**: Grilled Chicken with Barley and Roasted Vegetables
- **Snack**: Hummus with Veggie Sticks

Day 5

- **Breakfast**: High-Fiber Pancakes with Berries
- **Lunch**: Black Bean and Corn Salad
- **Dinner**: Eggplant Parmesan
- **Snack**: Fruit and Nut Trail Mix

Day 6

- **Breakfast**: Spinach and Mushroom Omelet
- **Lunch**: Roasted Veggie and Farro Bowl
- **Dinner**: High-Fiber Veggie Stir-Fry
- **Snack**: Almond Flour Cookies

Day 7

- **Breakfast**: Almond Butter and Banana Smoothie
- **Lunch**: Sweet Potato and Black Bean Chili
- **Dinner**: Quinoa and Black Bean Stuffed Sweet Potatoes
- **Snack**: Berry Smoothie

Grocery List for High-Fiber Week

- Rolled oats
- Almond milk
- Chia seeds
- Whole grain bread
- Avocados
- Quinoa
- Mixed berries
- Bananas
- Mixed nuts
- Spinach
- Kale
- Feta cheese
- Cherry tomatoes
- Cucumbers
- Red onions
- Bell peppers
- Lentils
- Black beans
- Sweet potatoes
- Salmon fillets
- Chicken breasts
- Zucchini
- Broccoli
- Carrots
- Apples
- Honey
- Almond butter
- Whole wheat flour
- Greek yogurt
- Maple syrup
- Eggs

- Parmesan cheese
- Marinara sauce
- Olive oil
- Canned tomatoes
- Vegetable broth
- Red lentils
- Coconut milk
- Various spices and seasonings

Low-Residue Weekly Meal Plan

Day 1

- **Breakfast**: Smooth Banana Oatmeal
- **Lunch**: Chicken and Rice Soup
- **Dinner**: Baked Cod with Carrot Puree
- **Snack**: Applesauce

Day 2

- **Breakfast**: Scrambled Eggs with White Toast
- **Lunch**: Mashed Potatoes with Grilled Chicken
- **Dinner**: Pasta with Butter and Parmesan
- **Snack**: Yogurt with Honey

Day 3

- **Breakfast**: Rice Porridge
- **Lunch**: White Rice and Steamed Fish
- **Dinner**: Rice and Ground Turkey Casserole
- **Snack**: Banana Pudding

Day 4

- **Breakfast**: Smooth Applesauce Pancakes
- **Lunch**: Carrot and Potato Puree
- **Dinner**: Baked Chicken with Rice
- **Snack**: Smooth Peanut Butter Cookies

Day 5

- **Breakfast**: White Bread French Toast
- **Lunch**: Soft White Bread Sandwich with Turkey
- **Dinner**: White Fish and Mashed Potatoes
- **Snack**: Plain Crackers with Cheese

Day 6

- **Breakfast**: Rice Flour Muffins
- **Lunch**: Rice and Egg Salad
- **Dinner**: Soft Tofu Stir-Fry
- **Snack**: Soft Baked Apples

Day 7

- **Breakfast**: Soft-Boiled Eggs with Toast
- **Lunch**: Mild Chicken Curry with White Rice
- **Dinner**: Simple Risotto
- **Snack**: Gelatin Dessert

Grocery List for Low-Residue Week

- White rice
- White bread
- White flour
- Chicken breasts
- Cod fillets

- White fish fillets
- Ground turkey
- Soft tofu
- Eggs
- Plain yogurt
- Almond milk
- Bananas
- Carrots
- Potatoes
- Zucchini
- Bell peppers
- Onions
- Garlic
- Chicken broth
- Beef broth
- Vegetable broth
- Apples
- Honey
- Peanut butter
- Mild cheese (e.g., mozzarella, cheddar)
- Butter
- Pasta
- Olive oil
- Canned tomatoes
- Gelatin dessert mix
- Plain rice cakes
- Sugar
- Cornstarch
- Vanilla extract
- Various spices and seasonings

6

Lifestyle Tips for Managing Diverticulitis

Managing Diverticulitis involves more than just adjusting your diet. Incorporating healthy lifestyle habits can significantly improve your overall well-being and help prevent future flare-ups. Here are some practical tips:

Stay Hydrated

- **Drink Plenty of Water**: Aim to drink at least 8 glasses of water a day to keep your digestive system functioning smoothly.
- **Limit Caffeinated and Sugary Beverages**: These can cause dehydration and irritate your digestive tract.

Exercise Regularly

- **Engage in Gentle Exercises**: Activities such as walking, yoga, and swimming can help maintain regular bowel movements and reduce stress.
- **Avoid High-Impact Exercises During Flare-Ups**: Stick to gentle activities to avoid putting extra strain on your digestive system.

Manage Stress

- **Practice Relaxation Techniques**: Meditation, deep breathing exercises, and mindfulness can help reduce stress and its impact on your digestive health.
- **Find Activities You Enjoy**: Engage in hobbies or activities that help you relax and unwind.

Eat Mindfully

- **Chew Your Food Thoroughly**: Take your time to chew each bite properly to aid digestion.
- **Eat Smaller, More Frequent Meals**: This can help prevent overloading your digestive system and reduce the risk of flare-ups.

Keep a Food Diary

- **Track Your Meals and Symptoms**: Recording what you eat and any symptoms you experience can help you identify foods that may trigger flare-ups.
- **Adjust Your Diet Accordingly**: Use your food diary to make informed decisions about which foods to include or avoid.

Stay Informed

- **Educate Yourself About Diverticulitis**: Understanding your condition can help you make better choices and manage your symptoms effectively.
- **Consult with Healthcare Professionals**: Regular check-ups with your doctor or dietitian can provide valuable insights and support.

7

Conclusion

Managing Diverticulitis is a journey that requires patience, understanding, and commitment. By following the recipes and meal plans in this cookbook, you can take control of your diet and significantly improve your quality of life. Remember, you're not alone in this journey. Many people have successfully managed their Diverticulitis by making simple yet effective dietary and lifestyle changes.

Take it one day at a time, listen to your body, and don't be afraid to seek help when you need it. With the right approach, you can enjoy delicious, nutritious meals and lead a fulfilling, healthy life.

Thank you for choosing the "New Diverticulitis Cookbook for Beginners." Here's to your health and happiness—let's get cooking!

www.ingramcontent.com/pod-product-compliance
Lightning Source LLC
Chambersburg PA
CBHW071843210526
45479CB00001B/272